FARMER GYM UNLOADED

Farmer Gym Unloaded is an 8-week conditioning program designed to enhance one's overall fitness. Through structured training consisting of weight-bearing, body-weight, and running-based exercises, the program challenges the whole body. The book anticipates that you will work out 4 days a week, perform a steady-state run 1 day a week, and rest 2 days each week. You will proceed through Farmer Gym Unloaded day by day, just as you would a daily calendar.

Built into each workout are mechanisms for making the workouts more or less challenging. You can increase the weight of the Kettlebell and Dumbbells as you become stronger. You can increase or decrease the amount of rest during your workout. Don't be afraid to kick up the intensity if you find that you aren't breathing heavily or feeling any exhaustion during the workouts. But, take as many seconds of rest as you need during these workouts in order to safely perform the remainder of a set, or the next round. Your goal should be to work out for the entire allotted time, even if that means taking longer rests between sets. Never push yourself without resting, at the expense of good form or breathing. It's always better to take a break and recover than to burn out and quit, or to lose your form and injure yourself. If after the workout you feel unchallenged, try increasing the weight or tempo the next time you perform it.

Each workout in Farmer Gym Unloaded includes its own Notes section, where you can jot down your performance and measure your progress. This will serve to help you not only learn about your body, but also be encouraged as you see your performance improve on the various exercises. If competition motivates you, then make it a competition against yourself (or a partner!), and keep score. For example: If after Week 1, Day 1 you perform the workout in 27:17, write it down. When you come back to this workout during Week 5, Day 1, attempt to better your time. Or, if after Week 3, Day 2 you finish the workout with 4.5 rounds, try to better that number when you come back to it during Week 7, day 2.

EQUIPMENT

A few things are needed to successfully use Farmer Gym Unloaded. They are as follows: Dumbbells, a Kettlebell, and an optional Pull-up bar. Both the Dumbbell and Kettlebell are great for building strength, power, stability, and cardiovascular endurance. Found in most gyms, the familiar dumbbell is a popular weight-bearing tool that requires the body to generate power, thus developing one's strength. A more novel piece of equipment, the Kettlebell, due to its weight and changing center of gravity during use, requires the body to exert force and maintain balance in a number of positions. Compared to large, fancy machines, these pieces of equipments are very inexpensive – plus, they can be stored out of the way and take up very little space. The best part, though? They can go anywhere.

How to choose the correct weight: Always err on the side of caution, and don't attempt to increase the weight too quickly. Start with lower weights and gradually increase the size of the Kettlebell and Dumbbells you are using. It's important to perform each exercise correctly before moving up in weight. In the book you will find suggested weight ranges, but it should be noted: some professionals recommend that females start with a weight between 10 and 20 pounds for Dumbbells and 15 and 25 pounds for Kettlebells, gradually increasing in weight; it's recommended that males start with a weight between 15 and 30 pounds for Dumbbells and 25 and 35 pounds for Kettlebells, gradually increasing in weight. If you can easily perform 20 repetitions for an exercise without becoming fatigued, you may want to increase your weight.

In addition to the Dumbbell and Kettlebell, the Pull-up bar is an optional tool used in the book. You can use a basic high bar or rod. More than likely, there is one in a nearby gym, park, or schoolyard.

Of course, if you have a gym membership and do not wish to invest in a Kettlebell, set of Dumbbells, and Pull-up bar, you can take Farmer Gym Unloaded with you and use the equipment provided there.

WORKOUT DURATION

The workouts in the book last roughly 20-30 minutes in length. This might surprise you, or even make you skeptical (especially for the shorter workouts). But research has shown that vigorous exercise sessions lasting just 20-30 minutes are very effective in achieving fitness results. This kind of high-intensity workout has been found to improve cardiovascular health, increase fat burning, and boost energy levels. And, because many of the Farmer Gym Unloaded workouts are designed to use a high number of repetitions and to take the muscles to fatigue, these workouts tear down the muscle fibers, which lead to muscle definition, strengthening, and hardening.

WHO IS THE PROGRAM FOR?

This book is not for beginners; we recommend you have at least a year's worth of experience in the weight room and with high-intensity training before using the program. Most of the exercises found here should be familiar to you; if they are not, we suggest working on them before proceeding. This book is not for those seeking to improve max-effort lifts. Although you will likely see increases in general strength, the workouts are not meant to improve 1-rep maximums. Farmer Gym Unloaded is for those who wish to increase overall fitness by challenging their personal bests and testing their physical limits. If you are searching for the "bulky" look or a "skinny" frame, this book is also not for you; designed to grow strong, healthy, long-lasting muscle, the book is geared toward an "athletic" look.

A WORD ON NUTRITION

A substantial part of health and wellness lies in proper nutrition. When an exercise regimen is adopted in conjunction with a healthful diet, the results are synergistic. Although nutrition is beyond the scope of this Farmer Gym Unloaded, Farmer Gym emphatically encourages healthy eating. **(You CANNOT outwork a bad diet!)**

WARM-UP AND COOL DOWN

Before beginning each workout, spend up to 5 minutes getting your heart rate up and your blood flowing through your muscles. You can do this by jogging or marching in place, walking briskly for a short distance, or doing some Jumping Jacks. When you complete each workout, spend a few minutes slowing your heart rate gradually by marching in place again or walking around the block, and then stretching.

THE FINE PRINT

Farmer Gym Unloaded and Farmer Gym do not provide medical advice. As with any exercise program, you should consult your physician before using it, especially if you face any of the following risk stratifications: have any pre-existing conditions that include but are not limited to a heart condition, pain in your chest from physical activity, dizziness or loss of consciousness when working out, bone or joint problems, or are taking prescription drugs. Farmer Gym workouts and this book are intended for adults age 18 and over.

In addition, see your physician if you are a female over age 55, are a male over age 45, have a family history of heart disorder, have been a cigarette smoker in the past half-year, have led a sedentary life, are considered obese, are hypertensive, have high levels of lipids in your blood, or have a form of diabetes or other metabolic disorder. Likewise, when you are

performing the Farmer Gym Unloaded workouts, if you experience unusual pain, or if something doesn't feel right to you...STOP. Getting fit does not require injuries!

Farmer Gym has structured the workouts in the program to limit back-to-back, repetitive muscle strain; however, there remains an extremely remote chance of excess muscle damage from overuse. If you begin feeling pain in your joints or experience unusual soreness or health issues, temporarily discontinue your exercise regimen and see a medical expert.

Results are not guaranteed. How much progress you see toward your fitness goals will depend on how often you exercise, how hard you push yourself while exercising, what your diet consists of, how active you are apart from working out, your genetic composition, and other factors. Working out with Farmer Gym Unloaded is an excellent start, but is not the only determinant of your health, fitness, and strength outcome.

Be smart. Stay hydrated by drinking water before, during, and after your workouts. Work out in a place that is a safe temperature. And if you begin feeling dizzy or light-headed, stop.

One more thing. It's important to conduct your workouts in places that allow for stable footing. If you are doing portions of your workouts outside of a gym, make sure your exercise location accommodates safety, by choosing a flat, even surface that is not slippery or rocky.

Enough with the disclaimers. Let's start growing hard bodies!

THE MOVEMENTS

AIR SQUAT

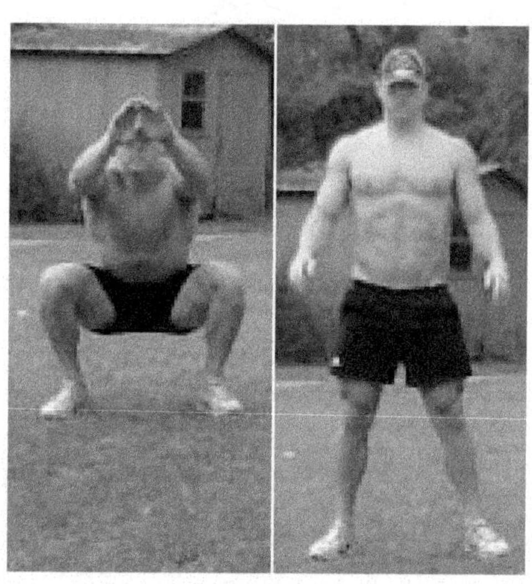

HOW TO: AIR SQUAT

* Stand with your feet at shoulder width and toes pointed slightly outward
* Keep your chest up, back straight, and core tight
* Descend by pushing your hips and gluteus back and down
* Keep your weight on your heels
* Stop once your thighs are at or below parallel to the ground
* Ascend by pushing through your heels
* Finish the squat in the starting position, standing up straight
* Your knees should not travel forward past your toes, nor should they turn inward

BURPEE

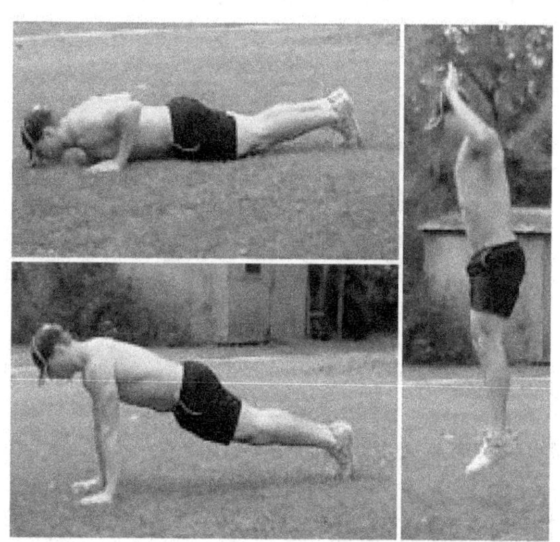

HOW TO: BURPEE

* Stand with your feet at shoulder width and toes pointed slightly outward
* Keep your chest up, back straight, and core tight
* With the weight on your heels, squat down and place your hands on the ground
* With the weight on your hands and shoulders, jump and extend your body until you are in a Plank-like position
* Descend until your chest touches the ground
* Push up and ascend to the Plank-like position, and jump your knees forward close to your chest
* Squat up, jump up into the air, and land in the starting position

(Scale: Perform the Push-up portion from your knees; perform without the Push-up)

CLEAN

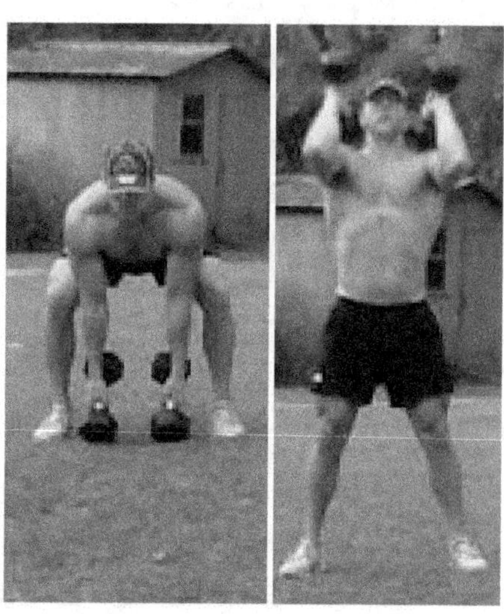

HOW TO: CLEAN

* Stand with your feet at approximately shoulder width and toes pointed slightly outward
* Keep your chest up, and keep your head aligned with a straight spine throughout the exercise
* While maintaining a neutral spine, with your chest up, bend from your hips and slightly from your knees to reach for the Dumbbells
* Your shoulders should remain upright and straight as you lower toward the ground, and will be over the balls of your feet at the bottom position
* Grasp the Dumbbells at the bottom, and while maintaining a tight core, explode through the ground, extending your hips and knees
* The Dumbbells should remain close to the body as they are pulled upward
* The arms will bend as the Dumbbells are guided to the shoulders
* The body should be in full extension with your elbows up upon receiving the Dumbbells
* In a controlled manner, lower the weight to the ground

DEADLIFT

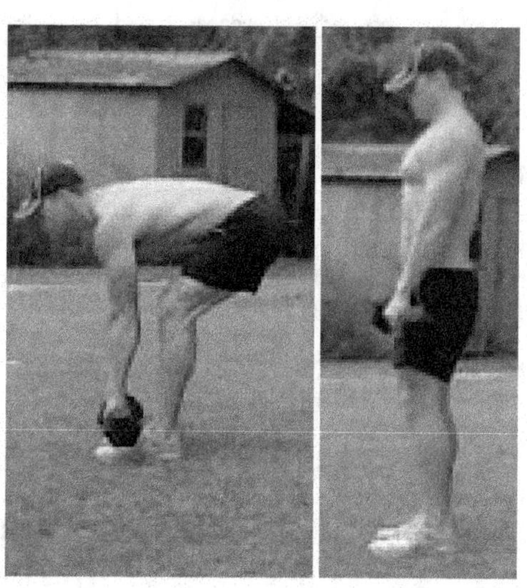

HOW TO: DEADLIFT

* Stand with your feet at approximately shoulder width and toes pointed
slightly outward
* Keep your chest and chin up, and keep your head aligned with a straight
spine throughout the exercise
* Bend your hips and knees at the same time, and In a controlled manner,
continue to bend your knees and shift your hips back and down on your
way down to pick up the Dumbbells
* Your shoulders should remain upright and straight as you lower toward
the ground, and will be over the balls of your feet at the bottom position
* Your knees should not travel forward past your toes, nor should they
turn inward
* At the bottom, grasp the Dumbbells, and while maintaining a tight core,
push your body up through your heels
* Your arms should remain straight, and the weights should stay close to
your body throughout the movement
* Ascend to the starting position by simultaneously straightening your
knees and hips
* Do not lower the weights beyond a position of mild stretch, and do not
bounce during the movement

(Scale: Substitute Dumbbells with the Kettlebell)

DOUBLE DUMBBELL ROW

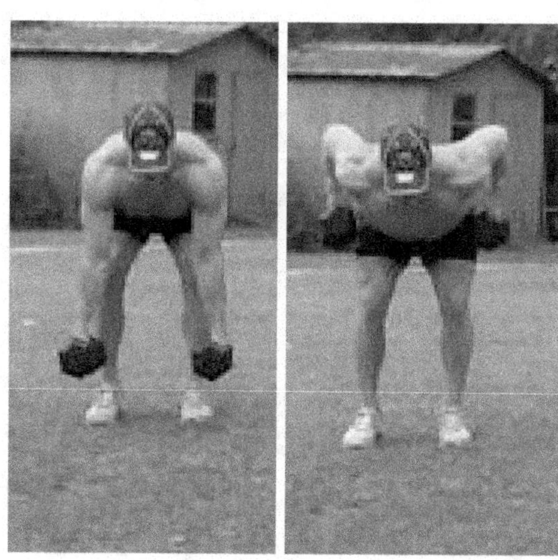

HOW TO: DOUBLE DUMBBELL ROW

* Stand over the Dumbbells with a hip-width stance, your knees slightly bent, and your mid-foot directly under the weights
* With your chest up, back straight, core tight, and hips elevated, reach down and grab the Dumbbells
* Contract your back, then drive your elbows back so that the Dumbbells reach chest level
* In a controlled manner, descend the Dumbbells by extending your elbows and returning the bar to the start position

DUMBBELL PUSH-UP

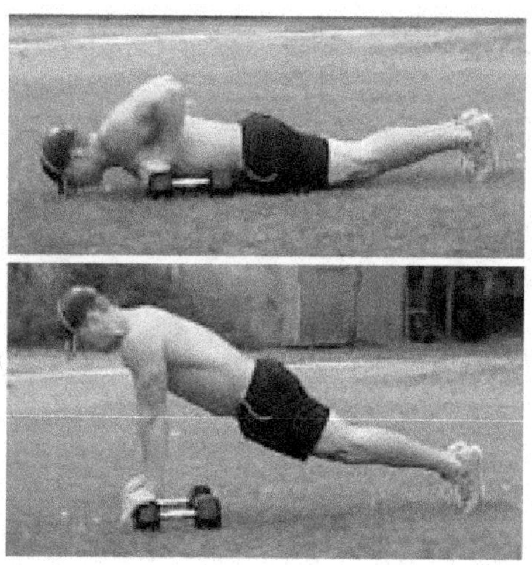

HOW TO: DUMBBELL PUSH-UP

* Lie face-down on the ground with your feet closer than hip-width apart
* With the Dumbbells lying next to your upper body, place the palms of your hands on the head of the Dumbbells, close to your shoulders
* With your toes on the ground and your elbows close to your side, push through your hands until your arms are extended
* Return to the ground slowly by bending your elbows until your chest reaches the ground

(Scale: Perform from your knees)

DUMBBELL ROW

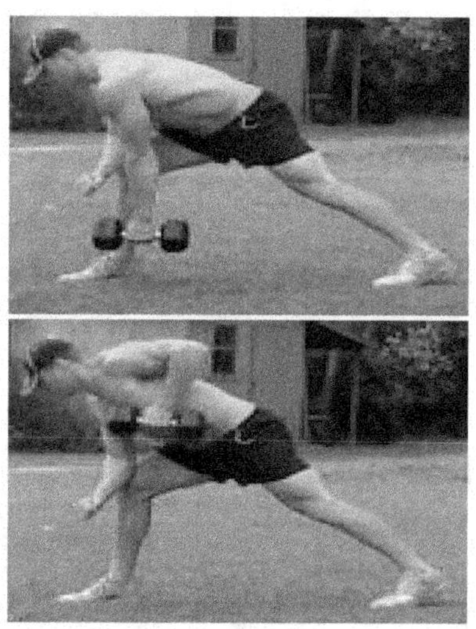

HOW TO: DUMBBELL ROW

* Stand while leaning forward with your chest up, with one leg in front of
the other and feet spread far apart
* Your front leg should be bent, and your front knee should not be past
your toes
* Your gluteus should be back, and your rear leg should be slightly bent
and facing forward
* The arm not engaged in the lift should rest on the front knee
* With your free arm, grab the Dumbbell and lift your shoulder first, then
your elbow, until the Dumbbell has reached your torso
* In a controlled manner, lower the Dumbbell back to the ground by
reversing the motion

DUMBBELL SNATCH

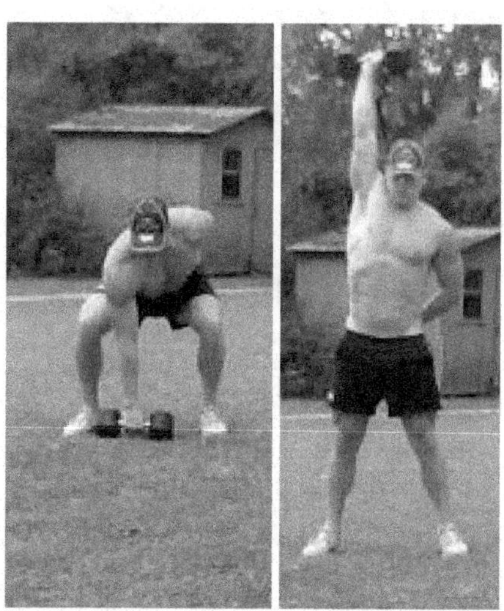

HOW TO: DUMBBELL SNATCH

* Stand with your feet shoulder-width apart and a Dumbbell between
your feet
* With your chest up and abs tight, grip the Dumbbell by slightly bending
your knees and shifting your hips back and down
* Press through the middle of your feet and drive the Dumbbell upward
* Keep the Dumbbell in a straight line, close to your body
* As the Dumbbell moves upward, drive your elbow high until the
Dumbbell is overhead
* Catch the dumbbell at the top position with slightly bent knees, then
stand upright
* In a controlled manner, reverse the movement and return the Dumbbell
to the ground

FARMER'S WALK

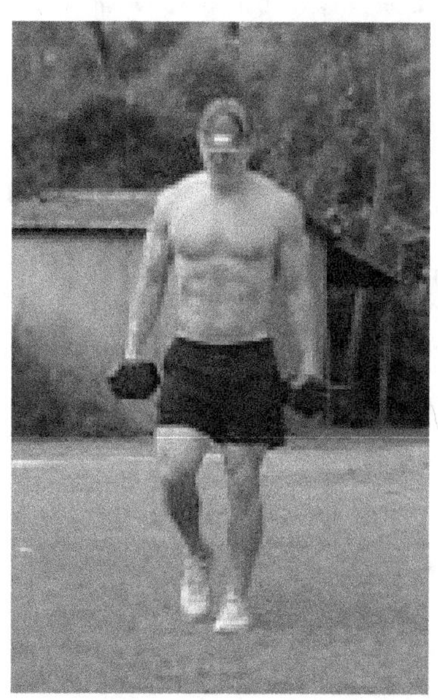

HOW TO: FARMER'S WALK

* Reach down to grab each Dumbbell, and then stand up with them
* Make sure your back is tight while grasping the Dumbbells
* With short, quick steps, walk with the Dumbbells while maintaining a
tight core

INVERTED ROW

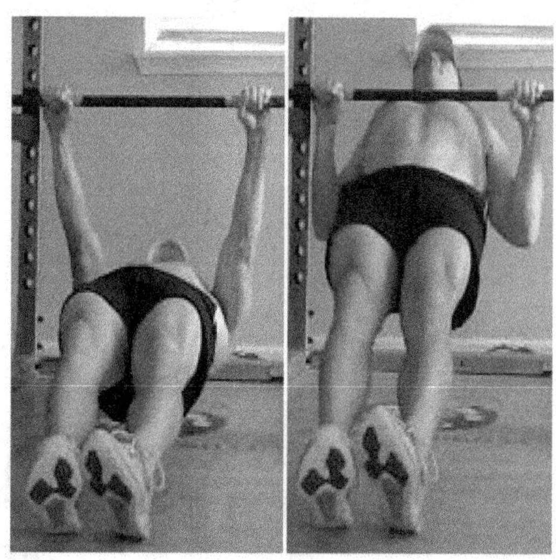

HOW TO: INVERTED ROW

* Position a bar around waist height, and make sure it's firmly in place
* Place your hands on the bar at wider than shoulder width while hanging underneath it
* Your body should be straight, with core tight, heels on the ground, and arms fully extended
* Pull your chest up toward the bar by bending your arms while maintaining a rigid body
* Pause once your chest meets the bar, then reverse the movement to descend to the starting position

JUMP SQUAT

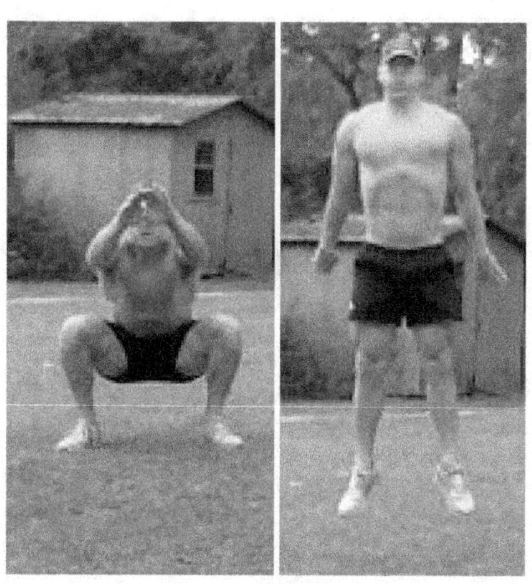

HOW TO: JUMP SQUAT

* Stand with your feet hip- to shoulder-width apart and toes pointed
slightly outward
* Keep your chest up, spine straight, and core tight
* Descend by pushing your hips and gluteus back and down
* Keep your weight on your heels
* Briefly stop once your thighs are parallel to the ground
* Explode by pushing through your heels then rolling onto the balls of
your feet, and jump into the air
* Softly land on the balls of your feet with your knees bent and feet
underneath your hips, and absorbing the force of the landing with your
hips

KETTLEBELL DEADLIFT HIGH-PULL

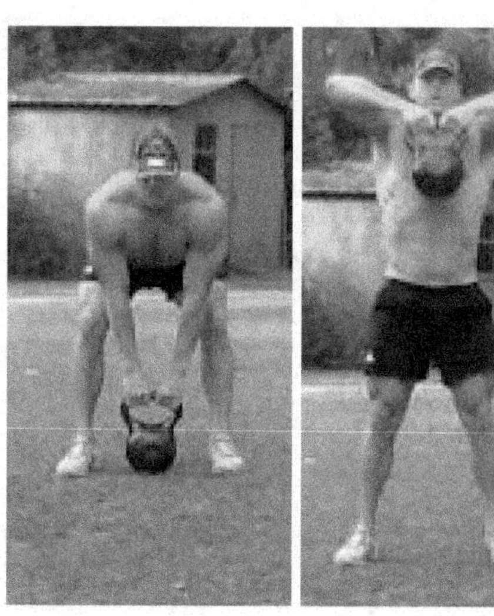

HOW TO: KETTLEBELL DEADLIFT HIGH-PULL

* Stand with your feet wider than shoulder width and toes pointed slightly
outward
* Keep your chest and chin up, spine straight, and core tight
* Descend by pushing your hips and gluteus back and down, without
letting your knees go past your toes or turn inward
* Keep your weight on your heels
* Grab the Kettlebell as you push through your heels and ascend to the
top; at about midway, pull the Kettlebell up toward your chin by flaring
your elbows out
* Keep your elbows held high once the Kettlebell reaches chin level
* Return the Kettlebell to the ground by reversing the ascension
movement

KETTLEBELL FRONT SQUAT

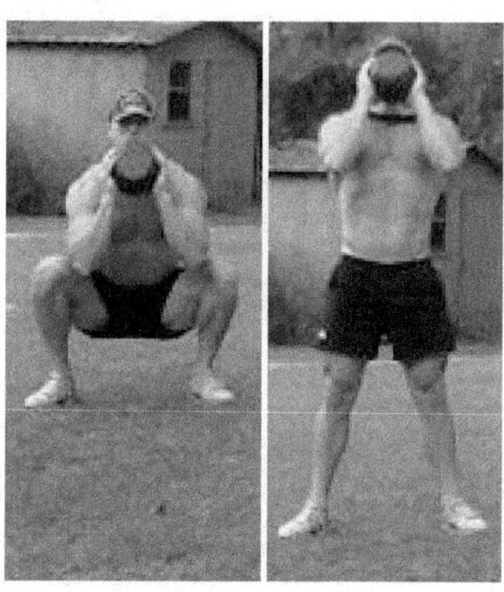

HOW TO: KETTLEBELL FRONT SQUAT

* Stand with your feet at shoulder width and toes pointed slightly outward
* Grab the Kettlebell by the handle with both hands, and hold it close to your chest with your elbows in
* Keep your chest and chin up, spine straight, and core tight
* Descend by pushing your hips and gluteus back and down
* Keep your weight on your heels
* Stop once your thighs are parallel to the ground, without letting your knees go past your toes or turn in
* Ascend by pushing through your heels
* Finish in the starting standing position

KETTLEBELL SQUAT PRESS

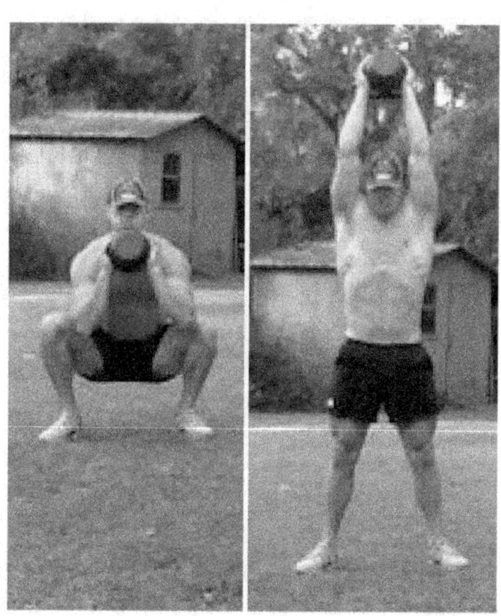

HOW TO: KETTLEBELL SQUAT PRESS

* Stand with your feet at shoulder width and toes pointed slightly outward
* Grab the Kettlebell by the handle with both hands, and hold it close to your chest with your elbows in
* Keep your chest and chin up, spine straight, and core tight
* Descend by pushing your hips and gluteus back and down
* Keep your weight on your heels
* Stop once your thighs are parallel to the ground, without letting your knees go past your toes or turn inward
* Ascend by pushing through your heels
* With your momentum, continue to drive the Kettlebell up and over your head, and lock your elbows out
* In a controlled motion, descend to the starting position

KETTLEBELL SWING

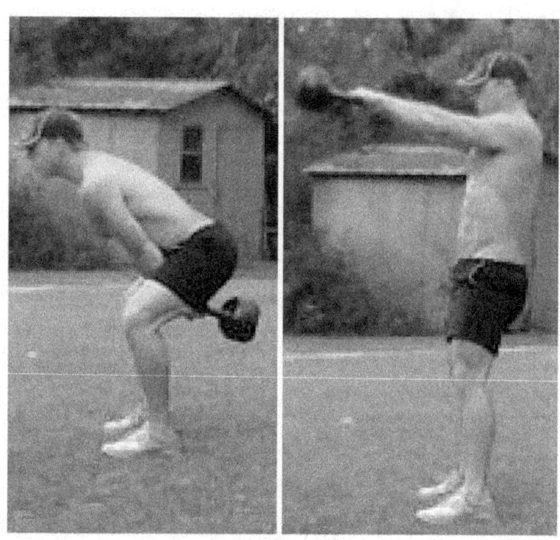

HOW TO: KETTLEBELL SWING

* Stand with your feet at shoulder width and toes pointed slightly outward, with the Kettlebell on the ground between your legs
* With your chest up and knees slightly bent, push your hips back and down
* Keep your weight on your heels
* Pull the Kettlebell close to your body and let it travel between the inside of your thighs
* Pop your hips and swing the Kettlebell forward
* Tighten your gluteus once your hips are open
* Let the Kettlebell use momentum and reach eye level
* Your arms should stay loose as the Kettlebell travels back to the starting position

LEG LIFT

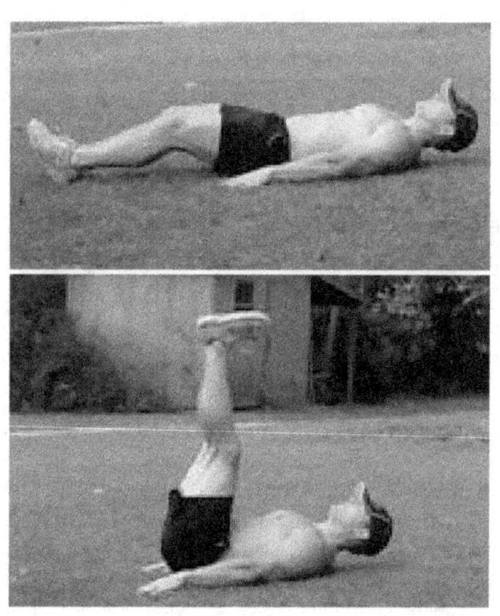

HOW TO: LEG LIFT

* Lie with your back and legs on the ground
* Place your hands under your lower back and gluteus
* With your feet together and legs straight, raise your legs off the ground
and bring them up until your toes are above your torso
* Slowly lower your legs until they are approximately an inch from the
ground

(Scale: Perform with bent knees)

LUNGE

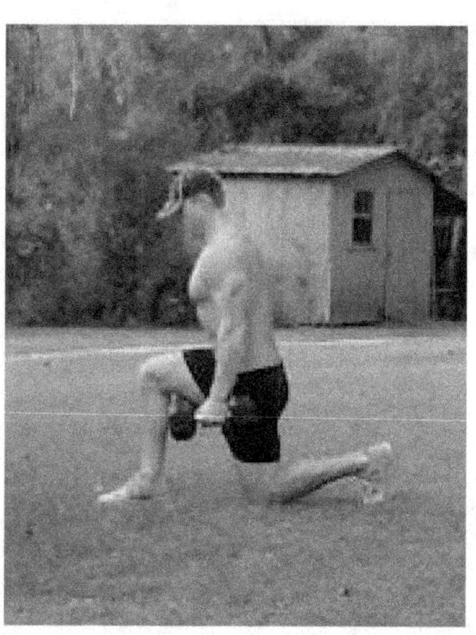

HOW TO: LUNGE

* Stand upright with your feet together (while grasping the Dumbbells)
* In a controlled manner, lift one leg off the ground and step forward
* Take a step, land with your heel first and toes pointing forward, and slowly shift the weight of your body onto your forward leg
* Maintain an upright torso, tight core, and straight spine
* Continue descending until your thigh is parallel to the ground, without letting your knee go past your toes
* Once in the lunge position, push off the front leg and return to the starting position, and alternate legs

MANMAKER

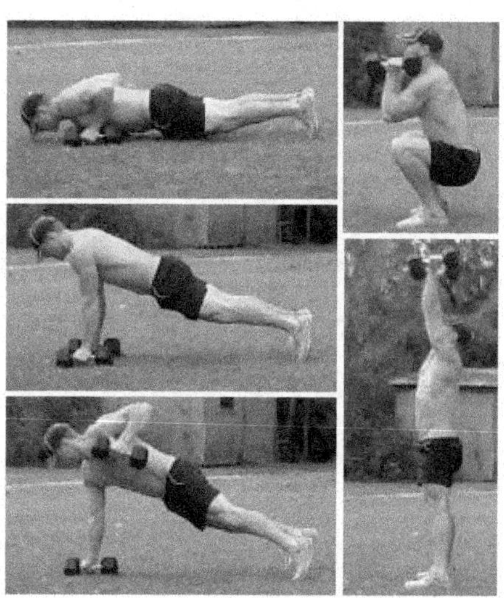

HOW TO: MANMAKER

* Lie face-down on the ground with your feet closer than hip-width apart
* With the Dumbbells lying next to your upper body, place the palms of
your hands on the head of the Dumbbells, close to your shoulders
* With your toes on the ground and your elbows close to your side, push
through your hands until your arms are extended
* While at the top of the Push-up, lift your shoulder, then your elbow,
until the Dumbbell has reached your torso
* In a controlled manner, lower the Dumbbell back to the ground by
reversing the motion
* With your opposite arm, lift your shoulder, then your elbow, until the
Dumbbell has reached your torso
* In a controlled manner, lower the Dumbbell back to the ground by
reversing the motion
* Then, while in the Plank-like position, jump your knees forward close to
your chest
* While keeping the Dumbbells at shoulder-level, squat up, and with a
tight core and straight back, drive the Dumbbells up and over your head
as you straighten your arms and press them into the air
* In a controlled manner, return the Dumbbells to the ground in a similar
manner as you lifted them

(Scale: Perform the Push-up portion from your knees; perform without
the Push-up)

OVER-THE-DUMBBELL BURPEE

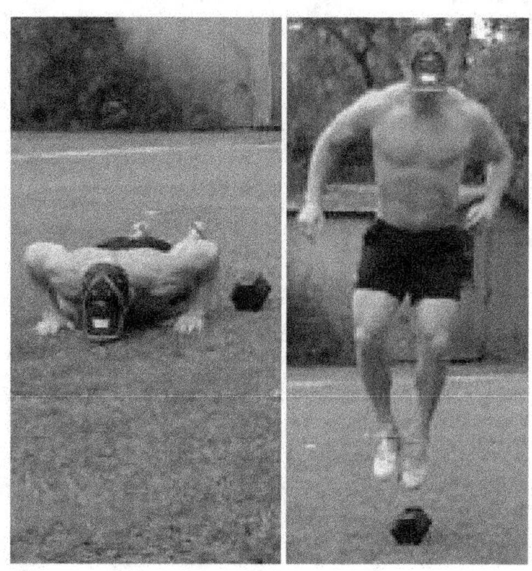

HOW TO: OVER-THE-DUMBBELL BURPEE

* Stand with your feet at shoulder width and toes pointed slightly outward
* Keep your chest up, back straight, and core tight
* With the weight on your heels, squat down and place your hands on the ground
* With the weight on your hands and shoulders, jump and extend your body until you are in a Plank-like position
* Descend until your chest touches the ground
* Push up and ascend to the Plank-like position, and jump your knees forward close to your chest
* Squat up, jump up into the air and over the Dumbbell, and land in the starting position

(Scale: Perform the Push-up portion from your knees; perform without the Push-up)

OVERHEAD PRESS

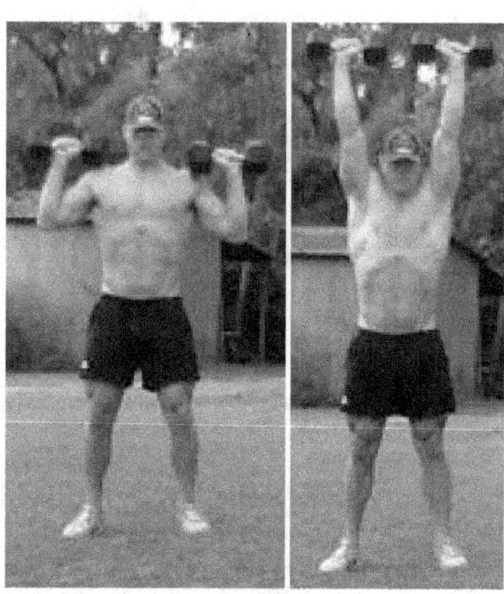

HOW TO: OVERHEAD PRESS

* Stand with your feet hip-width apart
* Hold the Dumbbells just wider than shoulder width
* Hold your wrists straight and keep your elbows close to your body and pointed downward
* With a tight core and straight back, drive the Dumbbells up and over your head as you straighten your arms
* In a controlled manner, reverse the movement and return the Dumbbells to the starting position

PULL UP

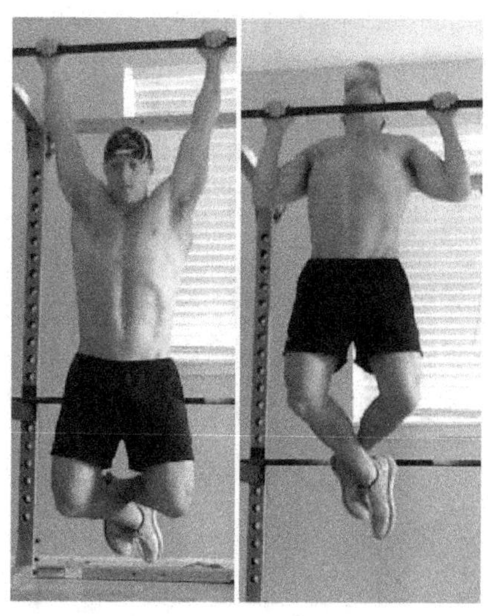

HOW TO: PULL-UP

* Hold the bar with your palms facing away from your body and hands
wider than shoulder width
* Keep your core tight, spine straight, and shoulders engaged
* Your head should be in line with your spine
* With both arms extended above you, pull your body up in a controlled
manner until your head is near bar level
* Upon reaching the top, slowly descend to the starting position

(Scale: Perform Lat Pull-downs if you have access to a gym; perform
Inverted Rows of Double Dumbbell Rows; for increased difficulty, perform
Pull-ups with added weight)

PUSH PRESS

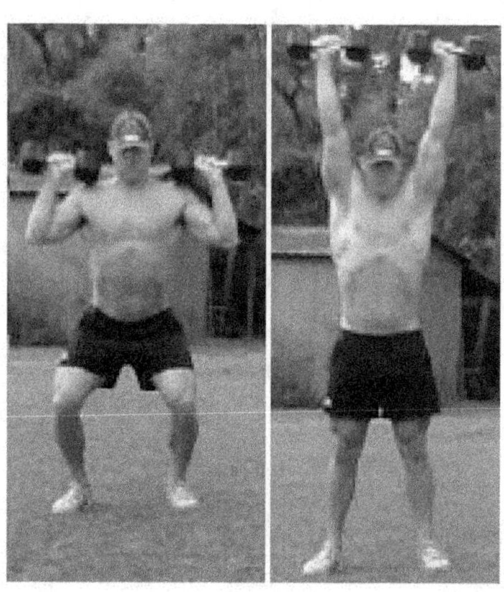

HOW TO: PUSH-PRESS

* Stand with your feet hip-width apart
* Hold the Dumbbells close to your body and just above your shoulders
* Hold your wrists straight and keep your elbows close to your body, with palms facing in
* With a tight core and straight back, slightly bend your knees and then press through the middle of your feet while driving the Dumbbells up and over your head as you straighten your arms
* In a controlled manner, reverse the movement and return the Dumbbells to the starting position

PUSH-UP

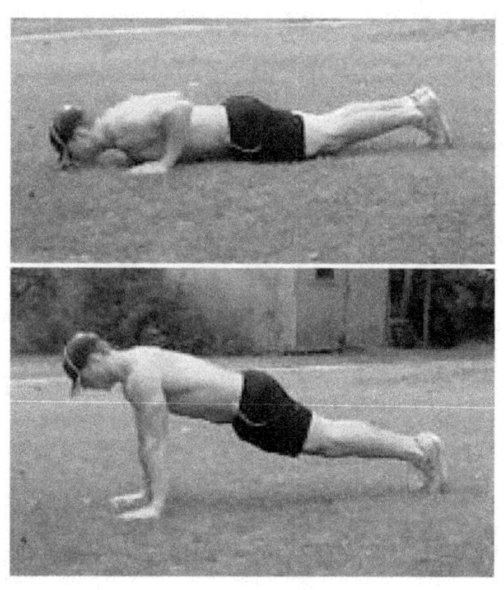

HOW TO: PUSH-UP

* Lie face-down on the ground with your feet closer than hip-width apart
* Place the palms of your hands flat on the ground, close to your shoulders
* With your toes on the ground and your elbows close to your side, push through your hands until your arms are extended
* Return to the ground slowly by bending your elbows until your chest reaches the ground

(Scale: Perform from your knees)

SIT-UP

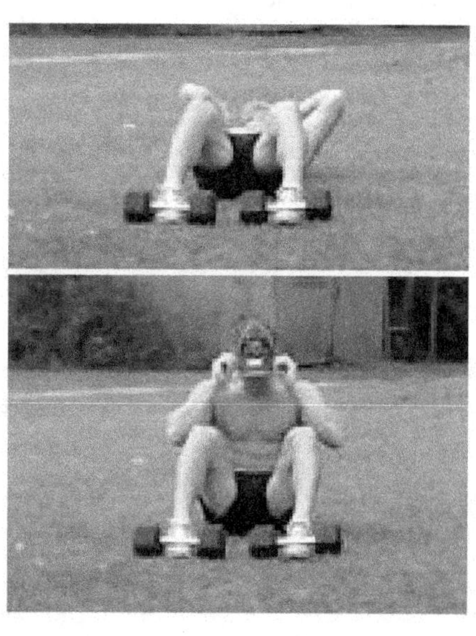

HOW TO: SIT-UP

* Lie down on your back with your knees bent and feet on the ground at hip width or slightly narrower
* With your elbows out wide, place your fingertips behind your head and squeeze your shoulder blades together
* With your gluteus and feet remaining on the ground, engage your stomach and raise your torso off the ground in a controlled manner until your torso has reached your thighs
* Descend by reversing the motion
* Keep your chin up and back straight throughout the exercise

(Scale: Perform the Crunch by raising your shoulders only a few inches off the ground)

TUCK JUMP

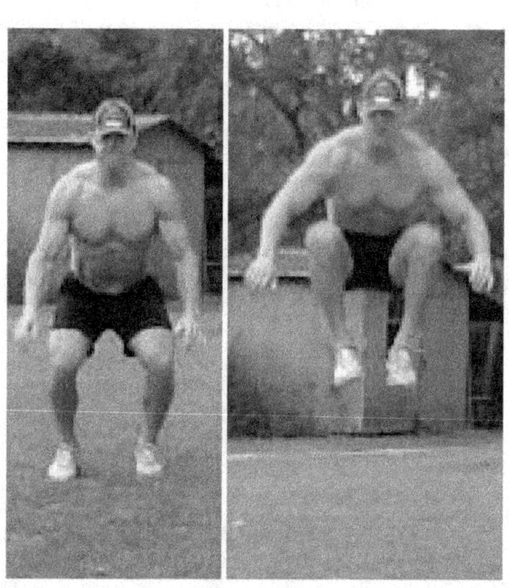

HOW TO: TUCK JUMP

* Stand with your feet at hip width and toes pointed forward
* Keep your chest up and core tight
* Reach your arms down as you bend at your hips
* After you descend to approximately the half-squat position, swing your arms up and jump straight into the air
* While in the air, tuck your knees into your chest
* Land on the balls of your feet, with your knees bent, weight somewhat forward, and chest up
* Immediately spring back into the air and repeat the motion

THE PROGRAM

<u>**Week 1, Day 1**</u>

The Workout:
(4 Rounds)
25 Manmakers
400-meter Run

*There is a 30-minute time cap.

Suggested male Dumbbell weight: 15-30#/Other#
Suggested female Dumbbell weight: 5-15#/Other#

Date	___/___/___	___/___/___	___/___/___
Time Performed			
Dumbbell Weight			

Notes:

<u>**Week 1, Day 2**</u>

The Workout:
50 Dumbbell Snatches (25 per side; alternate left to right)
50 Sit-ups
40 Dumbbell Snatches (20 per side; alternate left to right)
40 Sit-ups
30 Dumbbell Snatches (15 per side; alternate left to right)
30 Sit-ups
20 Dumbbell Snatches (10 per side; alternate left to right)
20 Sit-ups
10 Dumbbell Snatches (5 per side; alternate left to right)
10 Sit-ups

*There is a 30-minute time cap.

Suggested male Dumbbell weight: 30-70#/Other#
Suggested female Dumbbell weight: 10-45#/Other#

Date	__ / / __	__ / / __	__ / / __
Time Performed			
Dumbbell Weight			

(2-minute Rest)

3-minute Jump Squats

JS Performed			

Notes:

Week 1, Day 3

REST

<u>**Week 1, Day 4**</u>

The Workout:
(4 Rounds)
90-second Burpee
90-second Pull-up (Scale: Inverted Row; Double Dumbbell Row)
90-second Push-up
(90-second Rest)

If you scale with Double Dumbbell Rows, we suggested you use a weight that can be performed for no more than 15-20 reps in a row.

Date	___/___/___	___/___/___	___/___/___
Burpees Performed			
Pull-ups Performed			
(Scaled Performed)			
Push-Ups Performed			
Total Repetitions			
(Scaled Weight)			

Notes:

<u>**Week 1, Day 5**</u>

The Workout:
50 Kettlebell Squatpresses
1-mile Run
50 Kettlebell Squatpresses

*There is a 30-minute time cap.

Suggested male Kettlebell weight: 35-55#/Other#
Suggested female Kettlebell weight: 15-35#/Other#

Date	___/___/___	___/___/___	___/___/___
Time Performed			
Kettlebell Weight			

Notes:

<u>**Week 1, Day 6**</u>

20-minute Run

Date	___/___/___	___/___/___	___/___/___
Distance Run			

Notes:

<u>**Week 1, Day 7**</u>

REST

<u>**Week 2, Day 1**</u>

The Workout:
(3 Rounds)
Perform as many Pull-ups as possible in 2 minutes. There is a 15 Kettlebell Swing penalty every time you come off the bar. After the 2 minutes, you have up to 6 minutes to Run 800 meters. Once the 800-meter Run is complete, rest the remainder of the 6 minutes. (If running 800 meters takes too much time – more than 6 minutes – Run 400 meters instead.)

For example: Jane performs 7 Pull-ups, then comes off the bar for a brief rest. Before Jane can execute more Pull-ups, she must perform 15 Kettlebell Swings. And so on and so forth, until the 2 minutes are up. Upon Pull-up—Kettlebell Swing completion, Jane Runs 800 meters. She finishes the Run in 4:30; therefore, she has a 1:30 rest. After the 6 minutes, she begins Round 2.

*Scale: Inverted Rows; Double Dumbbell Rows

Suggested male Kettlebell weight: 35-70#/Other#
Suggested female Kettlebell weight: 15-45#/Other#

If you scale with Double Dumbbell Rows, it is suggested that you use a weight that can be performed for no more than 15-20 reps in a row.

Date	___/___/___	___/___/___	___/___/___
Pull-ups Performed			
(Scaled Performed)			
Kettlebell Weight			
(Scaled Weight)			

Notes:

<u>**Week 2, Day 2**</u>

The Workout:
(5 Rounds)
Perform as many Push-ups as possible
(30-second Rest)
Run as far as possible in 3 minutes
(2-minute Rest)

Date	___/___/___	___/___/___	___/___/___
Push-ups Performed			
Distance Run			

Notes:

<u>**Week 2, Day 3**</u>

REST

<u>**Week 2, Day 4**</u>

The Workout:
(30 Minutes)
6 Dumbbell Lunges (each leg; alternate left to right)
12 Deadlifts (same weight as Lunge weight)
24 Leg Lifts
48 Jumping Jacks

Suggested male Dumbbell weight (each Dumbbell): 35-70#/Other#
Suggested female Dumbbell weight (each Dumbbell): 15-45#/Other#

Date	___ / ___ / ___	___ / ___ / ___	___ / ___ / ___
Rounds Performed			
Dumbbell Weight			

Notes:

<u>Week 2, Day 5</u>

The Workout:
(4 Rounds)
30 Push-presses
20 Over-the-Dumbbell Burpees
10 Dumbbell Rows (each side)
400-meter Run

*There is a 30-minute time cap.

Suggested male Push-press Dumbbell weight (each Dumbbell): 35-70#/Other#
Suggested female Push-press Dumbbell weight (each Dumbbell): 15-35#/Other#
Suggested male Dumbbell Row weight: 35-70#/Other#
Suggested female Dumbbell Row weight: 15-45#/Other#

Date	___/___/___	___/___/___	___/___/___
Time Performed			
PP Dumbbell Weight			
R Dumbbell Weight			

Notes:

<u>**Week 2, Day 6**</u>

2-mile Run

Date	___/___/___	___/___/___	___/___/___
Time Performed			

Notes:

<u>**Week 2, Day 7**</u>

REST

<u>**Week 3, Day 1**</u>

The Workout:
(4 Rounds)
Set your clock for 5 minutes, then perform 25 Kettlebell Deadlift High-pulls,
followed by a Run for the remainder of the 5 minutes. Rest 2 minutes in between
each round.

For example: John sets his clock for 5 minutes, then starts the timer. He performs
25 Kettlebell Deadlift High-pulls, then Runs as far as possible with the remainder
of the 5 minutes. Once the timer finishes, he rests 2 minutes. After the 2-minute
break, John starts the clock and performs round 2.

Suggested male Kettlebell weight: 35-70#/Other#
Suggested female Kettlebell weight: 15-45#/Other#

Date	___ / ___ / ___	___ / ___ / ___	___ / ___ / ___
Distance Run			
Kettlebell Weight			

Notes:

<u>**Week 3, Day 2**</u>

The Workout:
(30 Minutes)
7 Tuck Jumps
14 Manmakers
28 Sit-ups

Suggested male Dumbbell weight: 15-30#/Other#
Suggested female Dumbbell weight: 5-15#/Other#

Date	/ /	/ /	/ /
Rounds Performed			
Dumbbell Weight			

Notes:

<u>**Week 3, Day 3**</u>

REST

<u>**Week 3, Day 4**</u>

The Workout:
(30-minute EMOM – Every Minute On the Minute)
Minute 1: 10 Dumbbell Cleans
Minute 2: 10 Kettlebell Front Squats
Minute 3: 10 Pull-up (Scale: Inverted Row; Double Dumbbell Row)
Minute 4: 10 Dumbbell Cleans
Minute 5: 10 Kettlebell Front Squats
Minute 6: 10 Pull-up (Scale: Inverted Row; Double Dumbbell Row)
…and so on and so forth, until 30 minutes is complete.

For example: Joe starts his clock, then performs 10 Dumbbell Cleans; he then rests for the remainder of the minute. At the next minute, he performs 10 Kettlebell Front Squats; after the Kettlebell Front Squats, Joe rests the remainder of the minute. At the next minute, he performs 10 Pull-ups; after the Pull-ups, Joe rests the remainder of the minute. This minute-by-minute alternating process continues until 30 minutes is up.

Suggested male Dumbbell weight: 35-70#/Other#
Suggested female Dumbbell weight: 10-35#/Other#
Suggested male Kettlebell weight: 35-70#/Other#
Suggested female Kettlebell weight: 15-45#/Other#

If you scale with Double Dumbbell Rows, it is suggested that you use a weight that can be performed for no more than 15-20 reps in a row.

Date	__/__/__	__/__/__	__/__/__
Dumbbell Weight			
Kettlebell Weight			
(Scaled Weight)			

Notes:

<u>**Week 3, Day 5**</u>

The Workout:
50 Burpees

Date	/ /	/ /	/ /
Time Performed			

(5-minute Rest)

15-minute Farmer's Walk. Every time you put the Dumbbells down, there is a 15
Push-up followed by a 30 Leg Lift penalty.

Suggested male Dumbbell weight (each Dumbbell): 45-70#/Other#
Suggested female Dumbbell weight (each Dumbbell): 20-45#/Other#

Date	/ /	/ /	/ /
Distance Walked			
Dumbbell Weight			

Notes:

<u>**Week 3, Day 6**</u>

30-minute Run

Date	___/___/___	___/___/___	___/___/___
Distance Run			

Notes:

<u>**Week 3, Day 7**</u>

REST

<u>**Week 4, Day 1**</u>

The Workout:
20 Kettlebell Squat Presses
1 Pull-up (Scale: Inverted Row; Double Dumbbell Row)
18 Kettlebell Squat Presses
2 Pull-ups (Scale: Inverted Row; Double Dumbbell Row)
16 Kettlebell Squat Presses
3 Pull-ups (Scale: Inverted Row; Double Dumbbell Row)
...and so on and so forth, decreasing Squat Presses by 2 and increasing Pull-ups
by 1, until the sequence of 2 Squat Presses and 10 Pull-ups have been completed.

*There is a 30-minute time cap.

Suggested male Kettlebell weight: 35-55#/Other#
Suggested female Kettlebell weight: 15-35#/Other#

If you scale with Double Dumbbell Rows, it is suggested that you use a weight
that can be performed for no more than 15-20 reps in a row.

Date	___/___/___	___/___/___	___/___/___
Time Performed			
Dumbbell Weight			

Notes:

<u>**Week 4, Day 2**</u>

The Workout:
(30 Minutes)
As many Push-ups as possible (once you must rest, move on to the next exercise)
30 Sit-ups
400-meter Run

Date	___/___/___	___/___/___	___/___/___
Push-ups Performed			

Notes:

Week 4, Day 3

REST

<u>**Week 4, Day 4**</u>

The Workout:
(3 Rounds)
10 Dumbbell Deadlifts
10 Burpees
...after the 3 rounds:
400-meter Run, then...
(2 Rounds)
10 Dumbbell Deadlifts
10 Burpees
...after the 2 rounds:
800-meter Run, then...
10 Dumbbell Deadlifts
10 Burpees
1-mile Run

*There is a 30-minute time cap.

Suggested male Dumbbell weight (each Dumbbell): 35-70#/Other#
Suggested female Dumbbell weight (each Dumbbell): 15-45#/Other#

Date	___/___/___	___/___/___	___/___/___
Time Performed			
Dumbbell Weight			

Notes:

<u>**Week 4, Day 5**</u>

The Workouts:
Tabata 1: Overhead Press
(2-minute Rest)
Tabata 2: Double Dumbbell Row
(2-minute Rest)
Tabata 3: Sit-up
(2-minute Rest)
Tabata 4: Air Squat
(2-minute Rest)
Tabata 5: Run

How to: Starting at minute 0, perform the selected exercise for as many repetitions as possible in 20 seconds, followed by 10 seconds of rest. At the 30-second mark, perform the exercise again for another 20 seconds, followed by 10 seconds of rest. Repeat this process for a total of 8 times; therefore, you finish around the 4-minute mark.

Suggested male Overhead Press Dumbbell weight (each Dumbbell): 20-45#/Other#
Suggested female Overhead Press Dumbbell weight (each Dumbbell): 5-20#/Other#
Suggested male Double DB Row weight (each Dumbbell): 20-55#/Other#
Suggested female Double DB Row weight (each Dumbbell): 10-25#/Other#

Date	___/___/___	___/___/___	___/___/___
OP Performed			
Rows Performed			
Sit-ups Performed			
AS Performed			
Distance Run			
OP Dumbbell Weight			
Dumbbell R Weight			

Notes:

<u>**Week 4, Day 6**</u>

3-mile Run

Date	___ / ___ / ___	___ / ___ / ___	___ / ___ / ___
Time Performed			

Notes:

<u>**Week 4, Day 7**</u>

REST

<u>**Week 5, Day 1**</u>

The Workout:
(4 Rounds)
25 Manmakers
400-meter Run

*There is a 30-minute time cap.

Suggested male Dumbbell weight: 15-30#/Other#
Suggested female Dumbbell weight: 5-15#/Other#

Date	/ /	/ /	/ /
Time Performed			
Dumbbell Weight			

Compare today's results with Week 1, Day 1:

Notes:

<u>**Week 5, Day 2**</u>

The Workout:
50 Dumbbell Snatches (25 per side; alternate left to right)
50 Sit-ups
40 Dumbbell Snatches (20 per side; alternate left to right)
40 Sit-ups
30 Dumbbell Snatches (15 per side; alternate left to right)
30 Sit-ups
20 Dumbbell Snatches (10 per side; alternate left to right)
20 Sit-ups
10 Dumbbell Snatches (5 per side; alternate left to right)
10 Sit-ups

*There is a 30-minute time cap.

Suggested male Dumbbell weight: 30-70#/Other#
Suggested female Dumbbell weight: 10-45#/Other#

Date	___/___/___	___/___/___	___/___/___
Time Performed			
Dumbbell Weight			

(2-minute Rest)

3-minute Jump Squats

JS Performed			

Compare today's results with Week 1, Day 2:

Notes:

<u>**Week 5, Day 3**</u>

REST

<u>**Week 5, Day 4**</u>

The Workout:
(4 Rounds)
90-second Burpee
90-second Pull-up (Scale: Inverted Row; Double Dumbbell Row)
90-second Push-up
(90-second Rest)

If you scale with Double Dumbbell Rows, it is suggested that you use a weight that can be performed for no more than 15-20 reps in a row.

Date	___/___/___	___/___/___	___/___/___
Burpees Performed			
Pull-ups Performed			
(Scaled Performed)			
Push-ups Performed			
Total Repetitions			
(Scaled Weight)			

Compare today's results with Week 1, Day 4:

Notes:

<u>**Week 5, Day 5**</u>

The Workout:
50 Kettlebell Squatpresses
1-mile Run
50 Kettlebell Squatpresses

*There is a 30-minute time cap.

Suggested male Kettlebell weight: 35-55#/Other#
Suggested female Kettlebell weight: 15-35#/Other#

Date	___ / ___ / ___	___ / ___ / ___	___ / ___ / ___
Time Performed			
Kettlebell Weight			

Compare today's results with Week 1, Day 5:

Notes:

<u>**Week 5, Day 6**</u>

20-minute Run

Date	___/___/___	___/___/___	___/___/___
Distance Run			

Compare today's results with Week 1, Day 6:

Notes:

<u>**Week 5, Day 7**</u>

REST

<u>**Week 6, Day 1**</u>

The Workout:
(3 Rounds)
Perform as many Pull-ups as possible in 2 minutes. There is a 15 Kettlebell Swing penalty every time you come off the bar. After the 2 minutes, you have up to 6 minutes to Run 800 meters. Once the 800-meter Run is complete, rest the remainder of the 6 minutes. (If running 800 meters takes too much time – more than 6 minutes – Run 400 meters instead.)

For example: Jane performs 7 Pull-ups, then comes off the bar for a brief rest. Before Jane can execute more Pull-ups, she must perform 15 Kettlebell Swings. And so on and so forth, until the 2 minutes are up. Upon Pull-up—Kettlebell Swing completion, Jane Runs 800 meters. She finishes the Run in 4:30; therefore, she has a 1:30 rest. After the 6 minutes, she begins Round 2.

**Scale: Inverted Rows; Double Dumbbell Rows*

Suggested male Kettlebell weight: 35-70#/Other#
Suggested female Kettlebell weight: 15-45#/Other#

If you scale with Double Dumbbell Rows, it is suggested that you use a weight that can be performed for no more than 15-20 reps in a row.

Date	___/___/___	___/___/___	___/___/___
Pull-ups Performed			
(Scaled Performed)			
Kettlebell Weight			
(Scaled Weight)			

Compare today's results with Week 2, Day 1:

Notes:

<u>**Week 6, Day 2**</u>

The Workout:
(5 Rounds)
Perform as many Push-ups as possible
(30-second Rest)
Run as far as possible in 3 minutes
(2-minute Rest)

Date	___/___/___	___/___/___	___/___/___
Push-ups Performed			
Distance Run			

Compare today's results with Week 2, Day 2:

Notes:

REST

<u>**Week 6, Day 4**</u>

The Workout:
(30 Minutes)
6 Dumbbell Lunges (each leg; alternate left to right)
12 Deadlifts (same weight as Lunge weight)
24 Leg Lifts
48 Jumping Jacks

Suggested male Dumbbell weight (each Dumbbell): 35-70#/Other#
Suggested female Dumbbell weight (each Dumbbell): 15-45#/Other#

Date	___/___/___	___/___/___	___/___/___
Rounds Performed			
Dumbbell Weight			

Compare today's results with Week 2, Day 4:

Notes:

<u>**Week 6, Day 5**</u>

The Workout:
(4 Rounds)
30 Push-presses
20 Over-the-Dumbbell Burpees
10 Dumbbell Rows (each side)
400-meter Run

*There is a 30-minute time cap.

Suggested male Push-press Dumbbell weight (each Dumbbell): 35-70#/Other#
Suggested female Push-press Dumbbell weight (each Dumbbell): 15-35#/Other#
Suggested male Dumbbell Row weight: 35-70#/Other#
Suggested female Dumbbell Row weight: 15-45#/Other#

Date	___ / ___ / ___	___ / ___ / ___	___ / ___ / ___
Time Performed			
PP Dumbbell Weight			
Dumbbell R Weight			

Compare today's results with Week 2, Day 5:

Notes:

<u>**Week 6, Day 6**</u>

2-mile Run

Date	___ / ___ / ___	___ / ___ / ___	___ / ___ / ___
Time Performed			

Compare today's results with Week 2, Day 6:

Notes:

<u>**Week 6, Day 7**</u>

REST

<u>**Week 7, Day 1**</u>

The Workout:
(4 Rounds)
Set your clock for 5 minutes, then perform 25 Kettlebell Deadlift High-pulls,
followed by a Run for the remainder of the 5 minutes. Your goal is to Run as far
as possible. Rest 2 minutes in between each round.

For example: John sets his clock for 5 minutes, then starts the timer. He performs
25 Kettlebell Deadlift High-pulls, then Runs as far as possible with the remainder
of the 5 minutes. Once the timer finishes, he rests 2 minutes. After the 2-minute
break, John starts the clock and performs round 2.

Suggested male Kettlebell weight: 35-70#/Other#
Suggested female Kettlebell weight: 15-45#/Other#

Date	___/___/___	___/___/___	___/___/___
Distance Run			
Kettlebell Weight			

Compare today's results with Week 3, Day 1:

Notes:

<u>**Week 7, Day 2**</u>

The Workout:
(30 Minutes)
7 Tuck Jumps
14 Manmakers
28 Sit-ups

Suggested male Dumbbell weight: 15-30#/Other#
Suggested female Dumbbell weight: 5-15#/Other#

Date	/ /	/ /	/ /
Rounds Performed			
Dumbbell Weight			

Compare today's results with Week 3, Day 2:

Notes:

REST

<u>**Week 7, Day 4**</u>

The Workout:
(30-minute EMOM – Every Minute On the Minute)
Minute 1: 10 Dumbbell Cleans
Minute 2: 10 Kettlebell Front Squats
Minute 3: 10 Pull-up (Scale: Inverted Row; Double Dumbbell Row)
Minute 4: 10 Dumbbell Cleans
Minute 5: 10 Kettlebell Front Squats
Minute 6: 10 Pull-up (Scale: Inverted Row; Double Dumbbell Row)
...and so on and so forth, until 30 minutes is complete.

For example: Joe starts his clock, then performs 10 Dumbbell Cleans; he then rests for the remainder of the minute. At the next minute, he performs 10 Kettlebell Front Squats; after the Kettlebell Front Squats, Joe rests the remainder of the minute. At the next minute, he performs 10 Pull-ups; after the Pull-ups, Joe rests the remainder of the minute. This minute-by-minute alternating process continues until 30 minutes is up.

Suggested male Dumbbell weight: 35-70#/Other#
Suggested female Dumbbell weight: 10-35#/Other#
Suggested male Kettlebell weight: 35-70#/Other#
Suggested female Kettlebell weight: 15-45#/Other#

If you scale with Double Dumbbell Rows, it is suggested that you use a weight that can be performed for no more than 15-20 reps in a row.

Date	/ /	/ /	/ /
Dumbbell Weight			
Kettlebell Weight			
(Scaled Weight)			

Compare today's results with Week 7, Day 4:

Notes:

<u>**Week 7, Day 5**</u>

The Workout:
50 Burpees

Date	___/___/___	___/___/___	___/___/___
Time Performed			

(5-minute Rest)

15-minute Farmer's Walk. Every time you put the dumbbells down, there is a 15 Push-up followed by a 30 Leg Lift penalty.

Suggested male Dumbbell weight (each Dumbbell): 45-70#/Other#
Suggested female Dumbbell weight (each Dumbbell): 20-45#/Other#

Date	___/___/___	___/___/___	___/___/___
Distance Walked			
Dumbbell Weight			

Compare today's results with Week 3, Day 5:

Notes:

<u>**Week 7, Day 6**</u>

30-minute Run

Date	___/___/___	___/___/___	___/___/___
Distance Run			

Compare today's results with Week 3, Day 6:

Notes:

<u>**Week 7, Day 7**</u>

REST

<u>**Week 8, Day 1**</u>

The Workout:
20 Squat Presses
1 Pull-up (Scale: Inverted Row; Double Dumbbell Row)
18 Squat Presses
2 Pull-ups (Scale: Inverted Row; Double Dumbbell Row)
16 Squat Presses
3 Pull-ups (Scale: Inverted Row; Double Dumbbell Row)
...and so on and so forth, decreasing Squat Presses by 2 and increasing Pull-ups
by 1, until the sequence of 2 Squat Presses and 10 Pull-ups have been completed.

*There is a 30-minute time cap.

Suggested male Kettlebell weight: 35-55#/Other#
Suggested female Kettlebell weight: 15-35#/Other#

If you scale with Double Dumbbell Rows, it is suggested that you use a weight
that can be performed for no more than 15-20 reps in a row.

Date	___/___/___	___/___/___	___/___/___
Time Performed			
Dumbbell Weight			

Compare today's results with Week 4, Day 1:

Notes:

<u>**Week 8, Day 2**</u>

The Workout:
(30 Minutes)
As many Push-ups as possible (once you must rest, move on to the next exercise)
30 Sit-ups
400-meter Run

Date	___ / ___ / ___	___ / ___ / ___	___ / ___ / ___
Push-ups Performed			

Compare today's results with Week 4, Day 2:

Notes:

<u>**Week 8, Day 3**</u>

REST

<u>**Week 8, Day 4**</u>

The Workout:
(3 Rounds)
10 Dumbbell Deadlifts
10 Burpees
...after the 3 rounds:
400-meter Run, then...
(2 Rounds)
10 Dumbbell Deadlifts
10 Burpees
...after the 2 rounds:
800-meter Run, then...
10 Dumbbell Deadlifts
10 Burpees
1-mile Run

*There is a 30-minute time cap.

Suggested male Dumbbell weight (each Dumbbell): 35-70#/Other#
Suggested female Dumbbell weight (each Dumbbell): 15-45#/Other#

Date	___ / ___ / ___	___ / ___ / ___	___ / ___ / ___
Time Performed			
Dumbbell Weight			

Compare today's results with Week 4, Day 4:

Notes:

<u>**Week 8, Day 5**</u>

The Workouts:
Tabata 1: Overhead Press
(2-minute Rest)
Tabata 2: Double Dumbbell Row
(2-minute Rest)
Tabata 3: Sit-up
(2-minute Rest)
Tabata 4: Air Squat

How to: Starting at minute 0, perform the selected exercise for as many repetitions as possible in 20 seconds, followed by 10 seconds of rest. At the 30-second mark, perform the exercise again for another 20 seconds, followed by 10 seconds of rest. Repeat this process for a total of 8 times; therefore, you finish around the 4-minute mark.

Suggested male OP Dumbbell weight (each Dumbbell): 20-45#/Other#
Suggested female OP Dumbbell weight (each Dumbbell): 5-20#/Other#
Suggested male Double DB Row weight (each Dumbbell): 20-55#/Other#
Suggested female Double DB Row weight (each Dumbbell): 10-25#/Other#

Date	___/___/___	___/___/___	___/___/___
OP Performed			
Rows Performed			
Sit-ups Performed			
AS Performed			
OP Dumbbell Weight			
Dumbbell R Weight			

Compare today's results with Week 4, Day 5:

Notes:

<u>**Week 8, Day 6**</u>

3-mile Run

Date	___ / ___ / ___	___ / ___ / ___	___ / ___ / ___
Time Performed			

Compare today's results with Week 4, Day 6:

Notes:

<u>**Week 8, Day 7**</u>

REST

BONUS WORKOUTS!

(The following workouts are not meant to be executed in a particular order or at a specified time. They are not part of the Farmer Gym Unloaded program. Execute them as your body is ready and able to do the work.)

<u>**Bonus 1**</u>

The Workout:
(4 Rounds)
5 Minutes:
30 Kettlebell Deadlift High-pulls
30 Sit-ups
30 Kettlebell Squat Presses
30 Leg Lifts
(2-minute Rest)
**When you begin the next round, start where you left off.*

For example: Jessie sets her clock for 5 minutes, then starts the timer. She performs as many repetitions of the 30-30-30-30 sequence as possible. Once the timer finishes, she rests 2 minutes. After the 2-minute break, Jessie starts the clock and begins where she finished the last round, and performs round 2.

Suggested male Kettlebell weight: 35-70#/Other#
Suggested female Kettlebell weight: 15-45#/Other#

Date	/ /	/ /	/ /
Reps Performed			

Notes:

<u>**Bonus 2**</u>

The Workout:
(30 Minutes)
5 Pull-ups (Scale: Inverted Row; Double Dumbbell Row)
10 Dumbbell Lunges (5 per leg)
15 Push-ups
20 Kettlebell Swings

If you scale with Double Dumbbell Rows, it is suggested that you use a weight that can be performed for no more than 15-20 reps in a row.

Suggested male Dumbbell weight (each Dumbbell): 35-70#/Other#
Suggested female Dumbbell weight (each Dumbbell): 15-45#/Other#
Suggested male Kettlebell weight: 35-70#/Other#
Suggested female Kettlebell weight: 15-45#/Other#

Date	__/__/__	__/__/__	__/__/__
Rounds Performed			
Dumbbell Weight			
Kettlebell Weight			
(Scaled Weight)			

Notes:

<u>**Bonus 3**</u>

The Workout:
800-meter Run
Then:
100 Kettlebell Squat Presses
**Perform 5 Burpees at the beginning of every minute*
...once 100 Kettlebell Squat Presses have been completed:
800-meter Run

*There is a 30-minute time cap.

For example: Once Jake returns from the 800-meter Run, he begins Kettlebell Squat Presses. He performs as many reps as possible in the first minute. After the minute is up, he executes 5 Burpees, then begins performing more Kettlebell Squat Presses. At the top of the next minute he again executes 5 more Burpees. This process continues until 100 Kettlebell Squat Presses have been finished. Then Jake runs his final 800 meters.

Suggested male Kettlebell weight: 35-70#/Other#
Suggested female Kettlebell weight: 15-45#/Other#

Date	__/__/__	__/__/__	__/__/__
Time Performed			
Kettlebell Weight			

Notes:

<u>**Bonus 4**</u>

The Workout:
(3 Rounds)
10 Manmakers
20 Tuck Jumps
30 Kettlebell Swings
40 Push-ups
50 Air Squats

*There is a 30-minute time cap.

Suggested male Dumbbell weight: 15-30#/Other#
Suggested female Dumbbell weight: 5-15#/Other#
Suggested male Kettlebell weight: 35-70#/Other#
Suggested female Kettlebell weight: 15-45#/Other#

Date	/ /	/ /	/ /
Time Performed			
Kettlebell Weight			

Notes:

<u>**Bonus 5**</u>

The Workout:
(4 Rounds)
10 Dumbbell Cleans
10 Pull-ups *(Scale: Inverted Row; Double Dumbbell Row)*
10 Burpees
10 Kettlebell Front Squats
400-meter Run

*There is a 30-minute time cap.

Suggested male Dumbbell weight (each Dumbbell): 35-70#/Other#
Suggested female Dumbbell weight (each Dumbbell): 15-45#/Other#
Suggested male Kettlebell weight: 35-70#/Other#
Suggested female Kettlebell weight: 15-45#/Other#

If you scale with Double Dumbbell Rows, it is suggested that you use a weight that can be performed for no more than 15-20 reps in a row.

Date	__/__/__	__/__/__	__/__/__
Time Performed			
Kettlebell Weight			

Notes:

<u>**Bonus 6**</u>

The Workout:
(10 Rounds)
3 Tuck Jumps
6 Kettlebell Swings
9 Double Dumbbell Rows
12 Depth Push-ups
15 Sit-ups
18 Jumping Jacks

*There is a 30-minute time cap.

Suggested male Kettlebell weight: 35-70#/Other#
Suggested female Kettlebell weight: 15-45#/Other#
Suggested male Double DB Row weight (each Dumbbell): 20-55#/Other#
Suggested female Double DB Row weight (each Dumbbell): 10-25#/Other#

If you scale with Double Dumbbell Rows, it is suggested that you use a weight that can be performed for no more than 15-20 reps in a row.

Date	___/___/___	___/___/___	___/___/___
Time Performed			
Kettlebell Weight			
Dumbbell Weight			

Notes:

<u>**Bonus 7**</u>

The Workout:
(30-minute EMOM – Every Minute On the Minute)
Minute 1: 10 Dumbbell Snatches (5 per side; alternate left to right)
Minute 2: :30 Sit-ups
Minute 3: 10 Kettlebell Squat Presses
Minute 4: 10 Dumbbell Cleans (5 per side; alternate left to right)
Minute 5: :30 Sit-ups
Minute 6: 10 Kettlebell Squat Presses
...and so on and so forth, until 30 minutes is complete.

For example: Jenni starts her clock, then performs 10 Dumbbell Snatches; he then rests for the remainder of the minute. At the next minute, he performs 30 seconds of Sit-ups; after the Sit-ups, Jenni rests the remainder of the minute. At the next minute, she performs 10 Kettlebell Squat Presses; after the Kettlebell Squat Presses, Jenni rests the remainder of the minute. This minute-by-minute alternating process continues until 30 minutes is up.

Suggested male Dumbbell weight: 30-70#/Other#
Suggested female Dumbbell weight: 10-45#/Other#
Suggested male Kettlebell weight: 35-70#/Other#
Suggested female Kettlebell weight: 15-45#/Other#

If you scale with Double Dumbbell Rows, it is suggested that you use a weight that can be performed for no more than 15-20 reps in a row.

Date	__/__/__	__/__/__	__/__/__
Dumbbell Weight			
Sit-ups Performed			
Kettlebell Weight			
(Scaled Weight)			

Notes:

<u>**Bonus 8**</u>

The Workout:
20 Dumbbell Deadlifts
20 Over-the-Dumbbell Burpees
15 Dumbbell Deadlifts
15 Over-the-Dumbbell Burpees
10 Dumbbell Deadlifts
10 Over-the-Dumbbell Burpees
5 Dumbbell Deadlifts
5 Over-the-Dumbbell Burpees

Suggested male Dumbbell weight (each Dumbbell): 45-70#/Other#
Suggested female Dumbbell weight (each Dumbbell): 20-45#/Other#

Date	___/___/___	___/___/___	___/___/___
Time Performed			

(5-minute Rest)

Tabata 1: Manmaker
(2-minute Rest)
Tabata 2: Push-up

How to: Starting at minute 0, perform the selected exercise for as many repetitions as possible in 20 seconds, followed by 10 seconds of rest. At the 30-second mark, perform the exercise again for another 20 seconds, followed by 10 seconds of rest. Repeat this process for a total of 8 times; therefore, you finish around the 4-minute mark.

Suggested male Dumbbell weight (each Dumbbell): 45-70#/Other#
Suggested female Dumbbell weight (each Dumbbell): 20-45#/Other#

Date	___/___/___	___/___/___	___/___/___
MM Performed			
Push-ups Performed			

Notes:

www.ingramcontent.com/pod-product-compliance
Lightning Source LLC
Chambersburg PA
CBHW070810260726
48660CB00005B/1793